# *easy* massage

### any age • any place • any time

**Fiona Harrold**

*Consultant*
Marc Salnicki

*Illustrated by*
Juliet Percival

CONNECTIONS
BOOK PUBLISHING

A CONNECTIONS EDITION
This edition published in Great Britain in 2007 by
Connections Book Publishing Limited
St Chad's House, 148 King's Cross Road
London WC1X 9DH
www.connections-publishing.com

Text copyright © Fiona Harrold 1992, 2007
Illustrations copyright © Eddison Sadd Editions 2007
This edition copyright © Eddison Sadd Editions 2007

British Library Cataloguing-in-Publication data available on request.

ISBN 978-1-85906-219-7

1   3   5   7   9   10   8   6   4   2

The text in *Easy Massage* is from *Massage* by Fiona Harrold,
published by Connections Book Publishing (2000). The illustrations
are based on photographs by Sue Atkinson.

Phototypeset in Meta using QuarkXPress on Apple Macintosh
Printed in China

# Contents

Introduction                                      4

**HEAD-TO-TOE MASSAGE**                           8

Back                                             10

Backs of Legs and Buttocks                       22

Chest and Neck                                   38

Face and Head                                    48

Arms and Hands                                   60

Fronts of Legs and Feet                          72

**STIMULATING MASSAGE**                          86

**DE-STRESS MASSAGE**                           102

**SOOTHING HAND MASSAGE**                       120

ABOUT THE AUTHOR                                128
ABOUT THE CONSULTANT                            128

# Introduction

It is impossible to overestimate the power of touch. As babies, we need touch to survive and to learn how wanted we are, primarily through the quality of touch we receive from our parents. We form impressions and make decisions about ourselves, other people and life from this initial contact. As adults, loving touch is vital to our emotional and physical well-being, and we use touch as an effective means of giving comfort and reducing pain, without thinking of it as 'massage'. Massage is, in fact, the oldest healing art, and we now know that by helping us to relax, it has a phenomenal ability to redress the ravages of stress on the body.

There is mounting evidence that stress and unhappiness prevent the immune system from fighting disease efficiently. Conventional medical thinking acknowledges that stress is at the root of over 70 per cent of all illness, and professionals who take a more holistic approach would put this figure much higher. Massage helps to reduce stress and so prevent the onset of illness. It also brings our attention to the fact that we are under stress, enabling us to rectify the situation before further damage is done.

In this book I endeavour to provide you with a straightforward, easy-to-follow guide to getting to grips with your own healing touch, no matter how much or how little time you have to spare. Massage is a wonderful skill to have, and my wish is that you will soon enjoy giving it as much as your partner likes receiving it.

*How to use this book*
The book begins with a head-to-toe massage that will teach you how to work on the whole body. This sequence takes just over an hour to complete, depending on how long you spend on each stroke. However, it is divided into six sections, one for each part of the body, so that you may choose to focus only on certain areas if you or your partner wish.

This whole-body session is followed by three shorter sequences: a 30-minute routine that will stimulate the whole system; a 30-minute de-stress massage; and a 20-minute treatment to soothe aching hands. All three are ideal for when you are short of time, and the de-stress and aching hands routines can be performed without your partner having to undress. Each of these short massages is, in the main, made up of a selection of the strokes shown in the head-to-toe sequence, so it is advisable to learn the head-to-toe sequence first.

Each section within the head-to-toe treatment begins with an introduction explaining how massage can benefit that particular part of the body. Here, you can learn about the muscles you will be working on, along with the health conditions that can be eased by regular massage treatments.

Once you're familiar with the instructions given, you may wish to perform massage without stopping to consult the book mid-session. The wall chart shown on the inside of the book jacket provides a handy memory aid for the three shorter sequences. In case you need to refer to the book for the full instructions for any step, the page numbers are given on the chart. Whichever session you choose, practise the strokes in the order shown.

*Grounding*

Whatever the length of the treatment, completing your routine in a caring, sympathetic manner is of upmost importance and sets the seal on a good treatment. At the end of a massage your partner will be feeling very relaxed and possibly quite distant. It would be quite wrong and certainly counterproductive for them to get up immediately – their mind will be slow and an abrupt change of gear would probably lead to a headache. It is also very therapeutic for them to acknowledge and savour the waves of profound relaxation rippling through their mind and body. Grounding literally means bringing the awareness back to the feet, and simply involves holding the feet to the floor for a minimum of 20 seconds. Following this, leave your partner to relax for a few minutes.

### How does massage work?

Massage restores balance and harmony to a troubled mind and tense body, it helps us to feel better about ourselves and it leaves us with a fresh, optimistic view of life.

The human body is extraordinary in its capacity to renew and regenerate itself. Its own self-regulatory mechanism returns the body to a state of internal balance and harmony even after we stretch all its systems to cope with excessive pressures. Chronic, long-term stress inhibits this natural rebalancing. By constantly exploiting the body with unrelenting demands, we deprive it of the time and energy to repair and restore itself to harmony. Massage intervenes, allowing the body to carry out its own healing by regulating the actions of the autonomic nervous system.

Deep relaxation is intensely pleasurable. While in this quietened state, our body produces endorphins – hormones that relieve pain and induce feelings of contentment and even euphoria. In my experience, endorphins are more effective than any drug for pain relief.

### Preparation

How you prepare for a massage significantly influences how much you and your partner enjoy it. The room in which you carry out the treatment needs to be quiet, tranquil, clean and comfortable. Try to provide clean, warm, soft towels. Heat is extremely important. Your partner's body temperature will drop during the massage, so heat the room up well beforehand and keep a heater nearby in case you need to boost the temperature. Your partner's muscles will not relax if the air is chilly, and the effect of your massage will be completely undermined.

Always place towels over any area of the body you're not working on directly, particularly areas you have just massaged, as it's important to retain the muscles' warmth. Keep a lightweight blanket available too – most people feel more comfortable when they're not fully exposed.

The ideal surface on which to perform massage is a thick futon or duvet. Whichever you use, if you are using oil, cover the surface with towels to protect it. Check that you have to hand everything you are likely to need. This will include two large towels and a blanket, oil, tissues and relaxing music. Sympathetic light also contributes to setting the mood. A side light is ideal and a candle or essential-oil burner makes a lovely addition.

Before you begin any massage, take a few minutes to relax to ensure that you are free from tension and mental preoccupations. Once your partner is positioned ready for you to begin, quietly ask them to breathe gently, and to let their body sink into the mattress or duvet.

*Using oils*
Oil provides a smooth surface for the strokes. A good-quality organic oil such as almond, sunflower or grapeseed also nourishes the skin. To make a luxurious mixture, add 10 per cent of either jojoba, evening primrose, apricot kernel or wheatgerm oil. You will need to add about 50 ml vegetable oil to massage the entire body, although this will vary according to the size of your partner, the amount of body hair and the texture of their skin – dry skin literally drinks in the oil. Vegetable oil is referred to as a 'carrier' or 'base' oil, when it's used with essential oils. The natural herb and flower essences penetrate the skin very quickly and must never be used undiluted.

Make up enough oil for only one treatment as the oils start to lose their potency once diluted with vegetable oil. Store all your essential oils in dark bottles as light quickly destroys their properties.

The most pleasant way of applying the oil to your partner's body after making contact is to leave one hand on the body and slowly pour the oil over the back of the hand. Spread the oil onto the body with your other hand and effleurage it over the area. Use enough oil to allow you to glide smoothly over the area but not so much that you can't knead without slipping.

# head-to-toe massage

## FULL-LENGTH SESSION

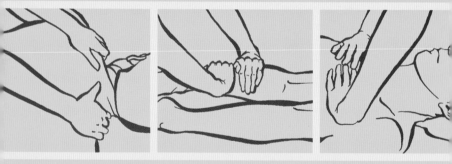

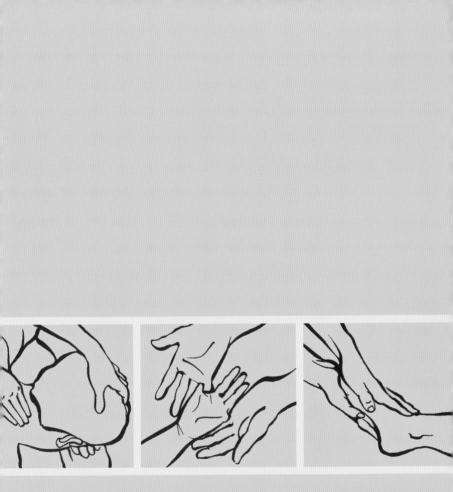

# back

The back is a wonderful area on which to give and receive massage. A good back massage will not only leave the back feeling relaxed and energized, but the whole body will benefit. This area is very vulnerable. Back pain accounts for more lost working days than any other complaint. Mental and emotional turmoil also lodges here. If only one part of the body is to be massaged, then the back is certainly the most effective.

Before you begin, ensure that your partner is in the correct position. You need to be able to reach the whole of this large surface area comfortably. Place your partner's arms out to their sides and kneel alongside them. Make sure you don't lean into their side: this will be uncomfortable and distracting for your partner. But, don't kneel too far away either, as you won't be able to work effectively.

## The Muscles Explained

The back is covered with large muscles, many of which connect the spine to the limbs. One of the largest of the back muscles is the trapezius, a flat muscle that extends from the base of the skull to the lower thoracic region of the spine and inserts into the shoulder blade. The trapezius is often a site of tension, causing discomfort in the neck, shoulders and upper back. The deltoid muscle connects the collar bone and shoulder blade to the humerus and makes the shoulder rounded. The teres muscles also onnect these bones. Lower on the back lies the latissimus dorsi.

**Caution: Do not massage the back if your partner has a slipped disc.**

*Eases pain across shoulder blades • Increases circulation of blood and lymph to the lower back following ligament injury • Relieves compression and lower-back distortion after pregnancy • Eases premenstrual tension • Benefits rheumatism sufferers*

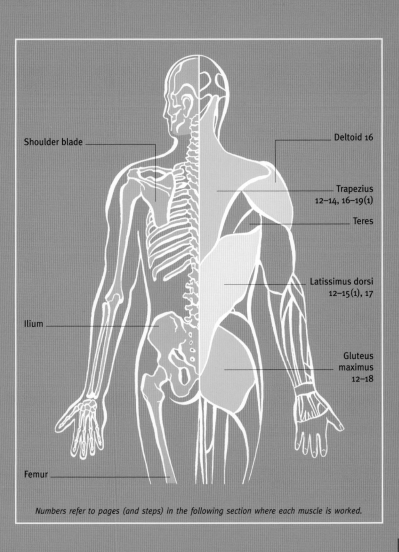

Shoulder blade

Deltoid 16

Trapezius
12–14, 16–19(1)

Teres

Latissimus dorsi
12–15(1), 17

Ilium

Gluteus
maximus
12–18

Femur

*Numbers refer to pages (and steps) in the following section where each muscle is worked.*

Apply oil to your hands, away from your partner's body. Breathe in, and, as you breathe out, make contact.

1 Glide both hands firmly up the back and around the shoulders.

2 Draw the hands lightly down the sides of the back to the starting position.

The dynamic here is on the upward motion towards the heart with light contact on the return stroke. Lean your body into your hands to apply more pressure. You can come up on your knees but keep the pressure steady. Repeat this four or five times.

Firmly stroking the body in this way is known as 'effleurage'.

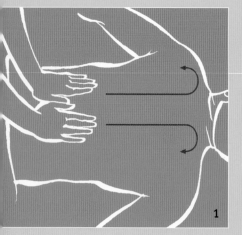
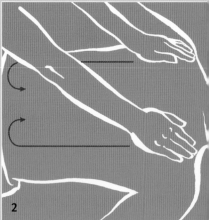

Glide your hands up the back once again.

1 Extend your hands over the shoulders, hook the fingers into the front of the shoulder muscles and pull back, leaning your body back for maximum effect.

2 The return stroke uses only the sides of the hands for very light contact, with the hands opened out.

Repeat twice.

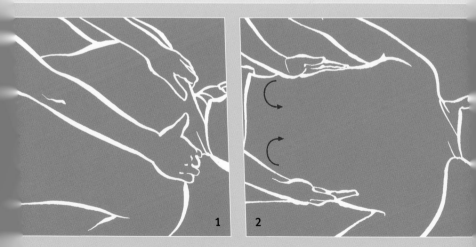

1  2

Place your hands on the lower back as if you are beginning to effleurage.

Push your hands out to the sides of the body, circling them around and back to meet each other. Continue the stroke, moving up the back with each set of circles until you reach the shoulders.

Draw the hands down to the lower back using the sides of your hands, as on page 13, step 2.

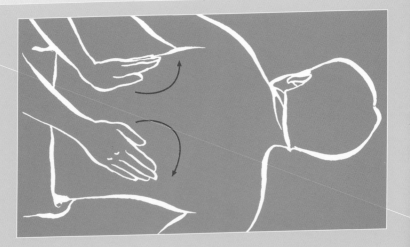

Place your hands on the lower back, fingers facing away from each other.

1   Lean the heels of your hands into the groove either side of the spine and begin to push towards your fingers. Do not allow the fingers to glide down the back. Work up the back to the shoulder blades, reducing the pressure as you cover the kidney area.

2   Repeat the stroke, working on one side of the spine at a time. Keep your hands parallel; rest one while the other works. You should work on the side furthest from you, so move round to the other side when you've finished one half. Work up to the shoulder blades. Squeezing the muscles in this way is called 'petrissage'.

Stay on this side to carry out the steps on pages 16–18 on one side of the back before repeating them on the other.

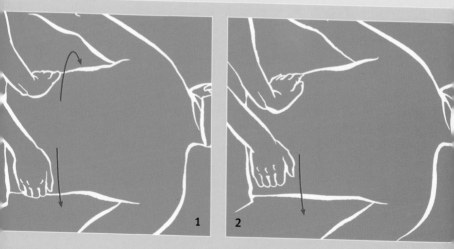

Check the position of your partner's arm, moving it gently if you need more room. Move your body so that your knees are facing your partner's back.

Begin to knead by pushing one hand into the muscle just below the armpit, picking up flesh and squeezing it between fingers and thumb. Then move the other hand in exactly the same way.

Set up an even rhythm with one hand starting as the other is finishing. Repeat four to five times.

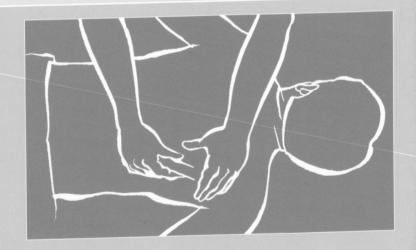

Move your knees to face the shoulder blade opposite.

1 Effleurage by placing both hands on the shoulder blade and pushing
   down towards the arm. Glide your hands in the direction of the arrows.
   Use your body weight to give momentum. When you push over the
   shoulder blade, come up onto your knees if necessary, but only if you
   can still control the pressure. Lean backwards using your full body
   weight when you pull the hands back.

2 To finish, rest your hands in opposite directions at the top of the
   shoulder blade.

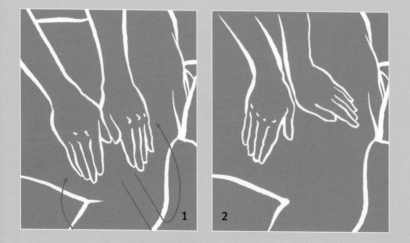

Return to your original position, kneeling alongside your partner.

Working on the nearest side of the body, place one hand on top of the other and, fingers straight and pointed, lean into the groove next to the spine. Slowly rotate the fingers on the muscle.

Work up the back, applying and releasing pressure very gradually, until you reach the shoulder. Continue in exactly the same way along the top of the shoulder, moving outwards from the neck. Repeat once.

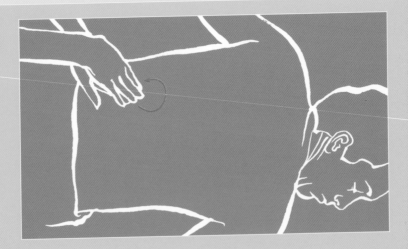

Ask your partner to rest their head on their hands. Position yourself comfortably with your body weight over the neck and head. Try placing your outside leg in front of you, foot parallel to your partner's head, inside leg kneeling up.

1   Stabilize the head with one hand while the other squeezes into the neck, working up towards the base of the skull. Don't let your thumb and forefinger slip around to the throat. Work up and down the neck three times.

2   Squeeze down the neck with one hand as the other squeezes up to meet it. Use your thumb and fingertips rather than the whole hand. Work up and down the neck three times.

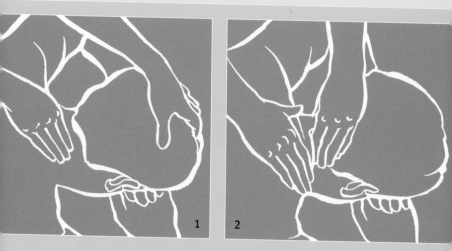

Effleurage again by leaning your hands into the lower back, gliding up to and around the shoulders, and down the sides of the body to the lower back. Repeat five times.

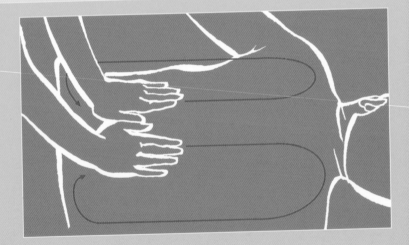

Beginning at the top of the back, draw your fingertips slowly down, one hand after the other. When one hand has reached the lower back, start at the top again.

Lighten the contact gradually to finish this stage, until your touch is almost imperceptible.

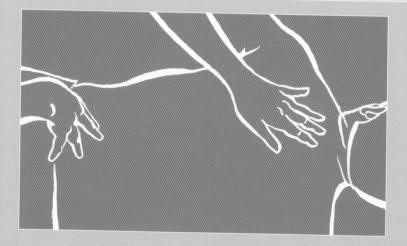

# backs of legs and buttocks

A sedentary lifestyle makes it hard for the blood and lymph to circulate around the backs of the legs. Gentle effleurage helps to reduce water retention in the ankles and thighs, and stimulates lymph flow in the backs of the knees and the groin. When massaging the backs of the legs, the distribution of your body weight is very important. Pressure on the calves should be applied sensitively and gradually, while on the backs of the knees it should be avoided completely. The thighs, however, require a very firm approach.

The buttocks are one of the most private parts of the body. It is the area least likely to receive touch. However, a great deal of tension is stored here, and it is a very pleasant area on which to receive a massage. Be especially confident in your touch. When applying petrissage (squeezing) strokes, work deeply and firmly.

Cellulite is a concern for many women. It occurs when the lymphatic system is unable to dispose of the toxins trapped between the tissues in fatty areas of the body, such as the buttocks and thighs. Combined with a healthy diet and exercise, massage is the only proven remedy for cellulite.

### The Muscles Explained

The gluteus maximus and the hamstrings are powerful, propulsive muscles. They lie across the back of the pelvis (the ilium portion of which is shown opposite) and the femur. The gluteus muscle forms the curve of the buttock and crosses the hip. The hamstrings cross the hip and knee. Below the knee, lying over the tibia and fibula, are the two bulky heads of the gastrocnemius or calf muscle. In the mid-calf region this muscle becomes the Achilles tendon, which then passes down to insert, finally, into the heel.

*Relieves cramp in the calf muscles • Eases cellulite and fluid retention • Eases pain caused by sciatica • Can prevent varicose veins*

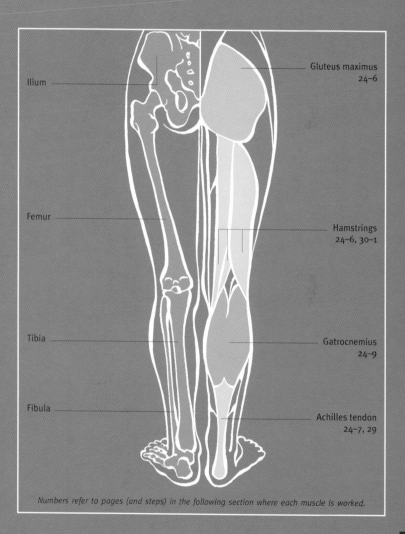

Ilium

Femur

Tibia

Fibula

Gluteus maximus
24–6

Hamstrings
24–6, 30–1

Gatrocnemius
24–9

Achilles tendon
24–7, 29

*Numbers refer to pages (and steps) in the following section where each muscle is worked.*

23

**Caution: Do not apply much pressure if your partner suffers from sciatica.**

Apply oil to your hands. Kneeling beside the feet, rest your hands gently on the leg, just above the ankle.

Inhale. Then, as you exhale, smooth your hands up the leg. Keep the pressure light, especially over the back of the knee. Reapply pressure once you have moved beyond the knee.

As your hands reach the top of the thigh, wrap your outside hand up and around the buttock in a smooth sweep, keeping the pressure firm. Be careful not to extend your inside hand too far up the inside thigh as this could feel invasive.

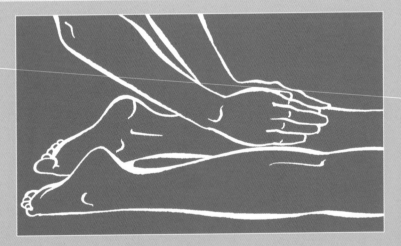

From the top of the thigh, draw your hands down the sides of the leg, keeping the pressure light. Remember to avoid any pressure on the back of the knee.

As you reach the calf, squeeze the muscle between the heels of your hands. Repeat this entire effleurage movement (pages 24–5) twice.

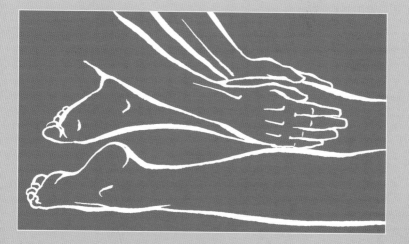

Place your hands on the lower leg in a cupped position, with your fingers pointing in opposite directions.

Breathe in, and, as you breathe out, lean gently into your hands, gliding them slowly up the leg. Ease the pressure as you reach the back of the knee, then reapply once you've cleared the sensitive area. Maintain the cupped position as you glide onto the thigh, and sweep firmly around the buttock with your outside hand.

Complete the stroke by drawing both hands lightly down the leg to the ankle.

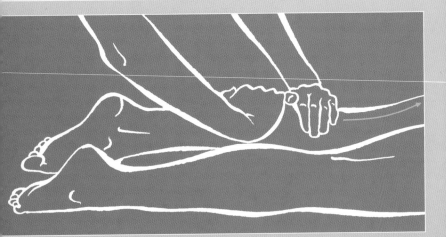

1 Place your hands flat on the lower leg. Breathe in, and, as you breathe out, push your hands up the calf as far as the knee. Here, pull your hands back to the ankle again. As you have already warmed the muscles with the opening effleurage strokes, you can now apply more pressure. Take the pressure off as you reach the back of the knee.

2 Wrap your hands around the calf, just above the ankle. Breathe in, and, as you breathe out, lean your weight into your hands to push up the calf as far as the knee. Lightly draw your hands down the sides of the calf to the ankle.

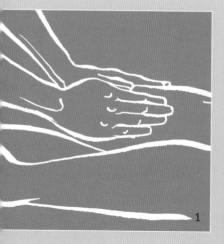
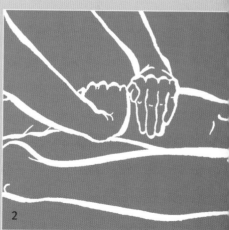

**Caution: Avoid petrissage, kneading and wringing strokes if your partner has varicose veins.**

Petrissage is the term used to describe any stroke that squeezes the muscles. Here, you are using the heels of your hands to squeeze the calf muscles.

Place both hands on the calf just above the ankle, the heels of your hands next to each other, fingers wrapped around the front of the leg.

Breathe in, and, as you breathe out, lean into the heels of your hands, pushing them away from each other and off the leg. Repeat this stroke moving up the calf until you reach the knee.

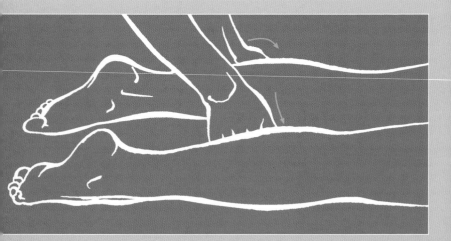

This time, you are using a wringing motion to squeeze tension and trapped toxins out of the muscles.

Reposition yourself to face your partner's calf.

1 Wrap your hands around the calf, embracing the muscles between your thumb and fingers. Use a firm wringing movement to lift and twist the muscles. Work over the entire calf.

2 Kneeling alongside the foot, rest one hand on the ankle. Wrap your other hand around the leg, resting your thumb on the centre of the calf. Inhale, and, as you exhale, lean slightly into your thumb and glide it up the centre of the calf to the knee. Apply very slight pressure to begin with. Repeat with your other thumb.

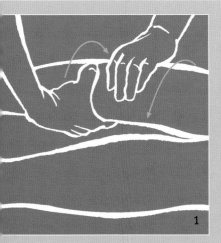
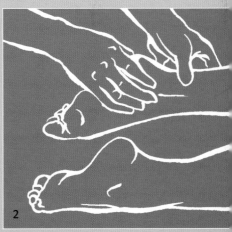

**Caution: Do not apply much pressure if your partner suffers from sciatica.**

Move further up the body to kneel by your partner's knees. Place your hands gently on the lower thigh.

Inhale, and as you exhale, lean your body weight into your hands and push up the leg. For extra weight, come up onto your knees, but keep your feet on the ground to ensure your pressure remains steady and secure. At the top of the thigh, turn your hands inwards and glide down to the knee. It's very important to respect your partner's privacy as you do this.

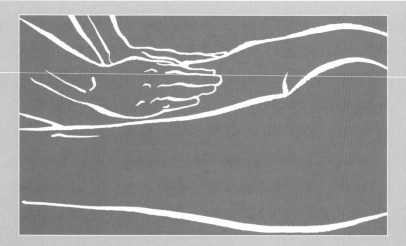

Cup your hands around the thigh.

Breathe in, and, as you breathe out, lean into your hands and push up the thigh. This feels great if you apply a lot of weight. At the top of the thigh push your outside hand up and over the buttock, maintaining the pressure, and pull it down the outside of the thigh, drawing your other hand down the inside at the same time.

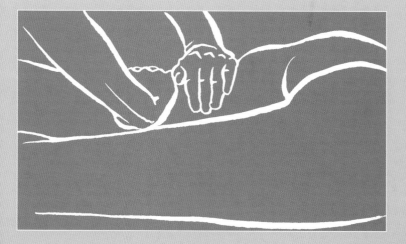

Make contact on the lower back.

Begin to effleurage the buttocks by gliding your hands away from each other, fingers pointing down towards the sides of the body. Draw the hands around the sides of the buttocks in the direction of the arrow. Push up over the buttocks and return to the starting position.

The pressure in this stroke is applied as you draw your hand around the sides of the buttocks and particularly as you push up and over towards the lower back. Repeat five times.

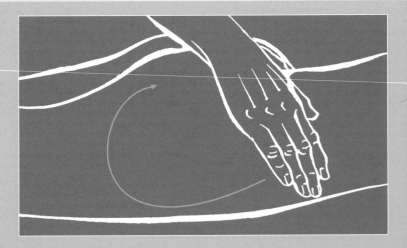

Move around your partner's body so that the leg and buttock you have been working on are furthest from you.

Still working on the same side, push one hand into the buttock, scoop up the muscle between your fingers and thumb and squeeze firmly. Repeat with the other hand.

Introduce a flowing rhythm by moving your hands alternately. Knead well all over the buttock.

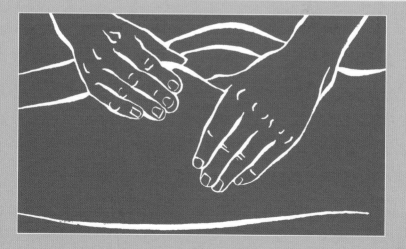

Beginning at the top, lean the heel of the hand into the buttock. As you push down, squeeze the muscle between the heel and fingers. Return to the top and repeat with the other hand.

Petrissage in this way five times with alternate hands.

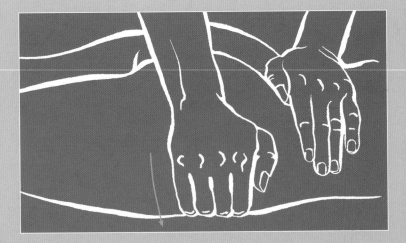

Next, we will be using some percussive strokes. Make the transition smooth by introducing gentle pummelling.

Bounce the hands alternately, moving over the entire buttock. Keep your hands close to the buttock at all times. Maintain an even pace, working faster only if you are able to keep to this rhythm. If you do speed up the stroke, check that your hands are still low.

Breathe deeply throughout this stroke; encourage your partner to do the same.

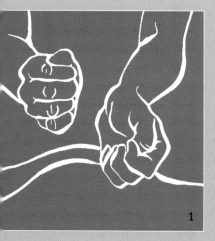
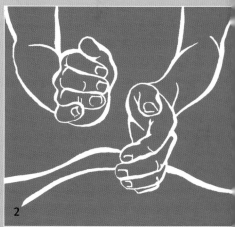

Place your hands on the buttock with one hand on top of the other, your fingers straight and relaxed.

Press your fingers into the muscles and rotate slowly. Aim to work deeply, but apply pressure according to your partner's tolerance. Work all over the buttock. It is imperative that you apply and release the pressure gradually, avoiding abrupt movements.

Repeat the entire sequence, from page 24, on the other leg and buttock.

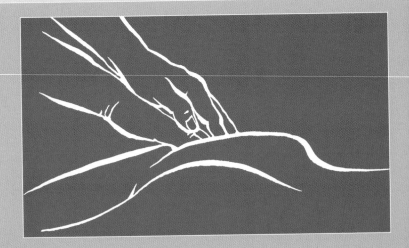

Effleurage by placing your hands on the lower back, gliding out to the sides, back towards you and pushing up over the buttocks. Start this stroke lightly, gradually applying more pressure, particularly as you push up over the buttocks. As you finish, lessen the pressure until your touch is as light as when you began. Repeat the stroke at least five times.

Effleurage at this point is particularly appreciated as it soothes the area after the deeper work and percussive stokes.

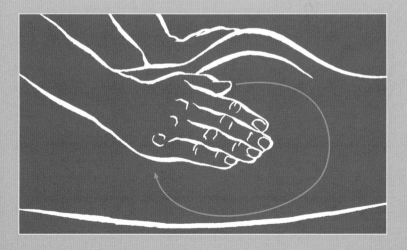

# chest and neck

The chest and neck are the most rewarding areas of the body to massage. Working directly on the skin with oil can feel so relaxing that your partner will feel like they have had a full-body treatment.

The head's position at the top of the spine is kept balanced by the co-ordinated action of the neck muscles. Problems often arise in this area if the head is held too far forwards, and this can lead to neck-and-shoulder strain and headaches. The upper chest can feel vulnerable when touched, as the heart and part of the lungs are housed here. Feelings of disappointment and sadness are stored and hidden in this area, as we see when someone sobs heavily and their whole chest heaves. Massage in this area can allow the recipient to feel safe enough to let go of their defences. In cases of emotional upset or trauma, a sympathetic touch on the upper chest can be enough to bring grief or sadness to the surface. Over time, massage will help relax emotional and mental armour, as well as that surrounding the body.

### The Muscles Explained

The pectoralis major is a broad, flat muscle that lies on the front of the chest wall and connects the ribcage, collarbone and humerus. The deltoid muscle is on the part of the shoulder furthest from the neck and works on the arm. The largest muscle, the trapezius, rises from the cervical and thoracic regions of the spine and connects to the base of the skull. Its fibres then spread out and insert into the shoulder blade. The trapezius supports the head and works the shoulders. Any tension here can spread to other areas.

*Eases aching pectoral muscles • Helps to relieve asthma • Eases the discomfort caused by wry neck*

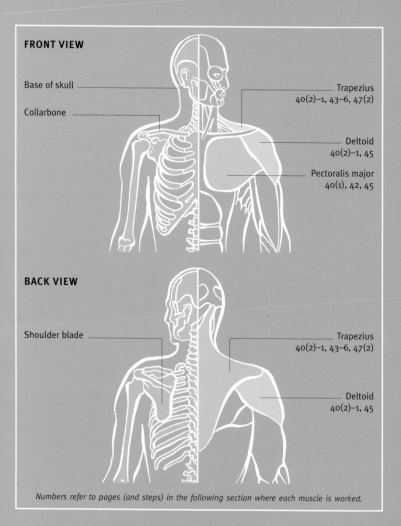

**FRONT VIEW**

Base of skull

Collarbone

Trapezius
40(2)–1, 43–6, 47(2)

Deltoid
40(2)–1, 45

Pectoralis major
40(1), 42, 45

**BACK VIEW**

Shoulder blade

Trapezius
40(2)–1, 43–6, 47(2)

Deltoid
40(2)–1, 45

*Numbers refer to pages (and steps) in the following section where each muscle is worked.*

**Caution: If your partner is suffering from asthma, apply gentle, mild strokes to the upper chest.**

Ask your partner to lie on their back. Position your knees astride the head. Apply oil to your hands.

1 Slowly and gradually, place your hands on the upper chest with your fingers facing each other. Don't lean into the chest; just rest the hands to establish contact. After at least 10 seconds, begin to effleurage by slowly gliding your hands away from each other, towards the shoulders. The pressure should be firm but not heavy.

2 Maintaining your position, wrap your hands around the shoulders. Increase the pressure and push the shoulders down. Keep your fingers closed and relaxed. Be flexible with your body, moving forwards slightly to increase the momentum in your hands.

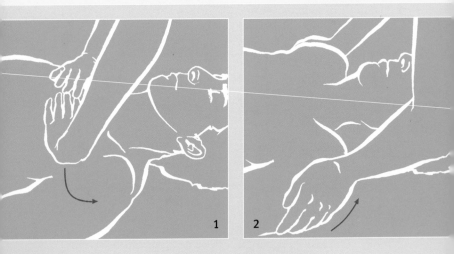

1 Scoop your hands under the shoulders and up underneath the neck until your fingers meet.

2 Cup the hands under the neck, and slowly pull towards you, leaning back so that the neck receives a gentle stretch. Draw the hands up to the base of the skull and gently release them.

Repeat the strokes shown on pages 40–1, three to five times. To finish, draw the hands up the back of the head, and off. Your intention here is not to lift the head but simply to continue the slow, gliding, stretching movement of your hands. Do this very slowly so your partner can fully relax their head.

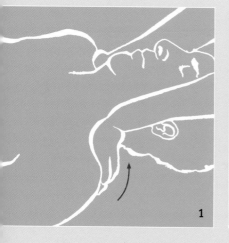

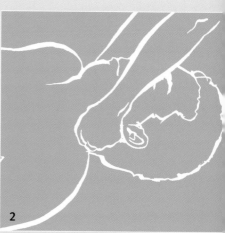

1 Form fists with your hands and place them on the upper chest. Rotate the fingers, moving them over the whole area and maintaining contact with the body. Work deeper into the fleshy areas in front of the armpits. This stroke feels wonderful when extended to the upper arms.

2 Rest one hand on your partner's shoulder while you work with the other hand. Lean the heel of this hand into the front of the pectoral muscle, next to the armpit. Anchor your hand by hooking your fingers underneath the muscle, and squeeze it between the heel and fingers. Then push your hand off the body. Repeat four times.

Rest this hand while you work on the other side. Be careful not to drag any hairs under the arms or on the chest.

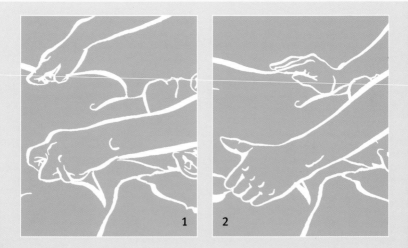

Using both your hands, gently and slowly turn your partner's head to one side. Allow the head to rest on your hand (the one nearest to the face).

Lean your free hand into the side of the neck and squeeze the muscles between your fingers and thumb. Work all the way along the neck, leaning your body weight into your hand for extra depth. Be careful not to let your thumb slide onto the throat.

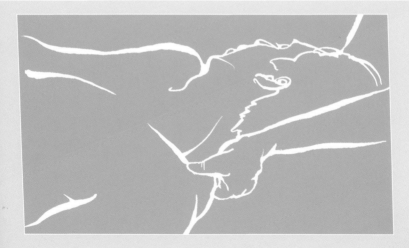

Place your hand at the top of the neck. Push into the neck, down and off at the shoulder. Bring your hand straight back to the starting position and repeat two to three times. Avoid the throat area, keeping your hand at the back of the neck and under the shoulders.

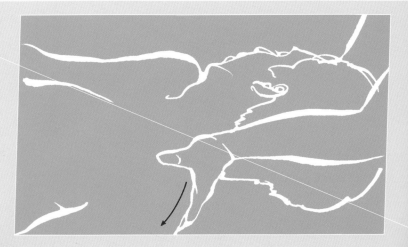

Keep your partner's head in the same position and place your hand on the chest below the collarbone.

1 Push into your hand and glide it across the chest, increasing the pressure as you move over the shoulder. Scoop the hand slowly around the shoulder, pushing it away from you.

2 Pull your hand very slowly up the neck, leaning your body back to increase the stretch. Take care to keep the hand to the back of the neck and avoid the ear. Continue the pull right up to and off the head. Repeat the step.

Turn the head carefully and repeat the steps shown on pages 43–5 on the other side.

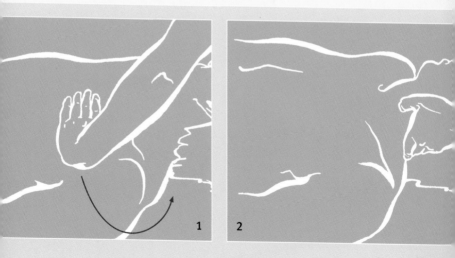

Gently and slowly, bring your partner's head back to a central position using both hands to support it fully during the movement. Rest one hand on the shoulder.

Place your free hand on the other shoulder, grasping the muscle with your thumb on top and fingers underneath. Lean your hand well into the muscle to get a more effective squeeze. Work thoroughly along the length of the muscle, making sure that the thumb doesn't slip onto the throat.

When you've finished working on one side of the body, rest the hand on the shoulder and repeat the stroke on the other side.

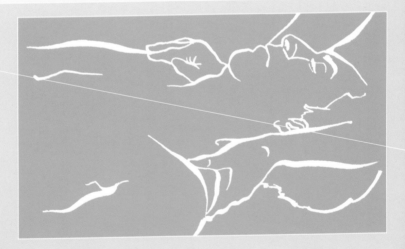

Place both hands on the chest.

1 Lean in and glide the hands across the chest, under the shoulders, up the back of the neck and off at the base of the skull.

2 Place the heels of both hands on the tops of the shoulders. Breathe in, and, as you breathe out, lean in to push the shoulders away from you, towards the feet – not down into the floor. It helps to lean forwards and down, without coming up onto your knees.

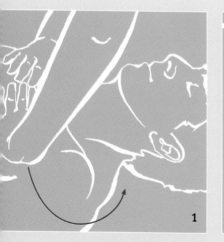

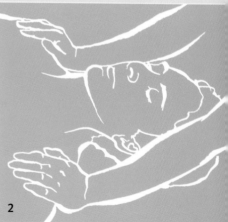

# face and head

The most exposed area of the body, the face reveals our thoughts and feelings. When we block our true emotions in favour of more acceptable ones, this conflict registers as tension in the facial muscles, which is a primary cause of premature ageing.

The muscles under the skin give the face its shape and contour. As they contract they cause the skin to wrinkle, and if the muscles remain tense this can be permanent. The most noticeable and immediate improvement you will see through massage is from the forehead strokes, which help to smooth out frown lines.

The face is the smallest, most sensitive area you will work on. You'll need to use your hands with greater dexterity and precision than you've done so far. A good facial massage can really improve the skin's health and appearance, boosting circulation and lymph flow, flushing out toxins and making the complexion glow. Try not to pull the skin as you work, as this could contribute to a loss of elasticity.

In the head there is a layer of muscle covering the skull, which tightens when we're tense and causes headaches. This can be loosened by massage, leaving your partner clear-headed and looking years younger.

### The Muscles Explained

The face contains a great number of muscles. The frontalis, zygomaticus and orbicularis muscles are concerned with producing facial expressions. The masseter is one of a group of muscles that moves the jawbone up and down during chewing. The ridge that can be felt just below the eyes is the cheekbone, which is attached to several facial muscles. The cranium comprises the bones of the skull.

*Eases headaches and symptoms of migraine • Reduces inflammation caused by sinusitis • Helps to improve blood circulation after a stroke*

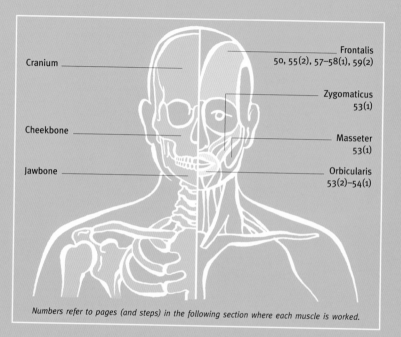

Cranium

Frontalis
50, 55(2), 57–58(1), 59(2)

Cheekbone

Zygomaticus
53(1)

Masseter
53(1)

Jawbone

Orbicularis
53(2)–54(1)

*Numbers refer to pages (and steps) in the following section where each muscle is worked.*

Kneel astride your partner's head. Rest your hands on the forehead, placing your thumbs in the centre and wrapping your fingers around the sides.

1   Inhale. Exhale and lean forwards slightly, transferring your weight into your thumbs. Glide them towards the ears, keeping them relaxed but straight, using even pressure along their entire length. When you reach the ears, place your thumbs back on the forehead, just above the original position. Repeat, moving upwards each time until you reach the hairline.

2   Rest the thumbs on the eyebrows. Inhale. Exhale and lean forwards to transfer weight into your thumbs. Draw them slowly across the eyebrows and down to the ears. Lift the hands, return to your starting position and repeat. Ask your partner what amount of pressure they find comfortable.

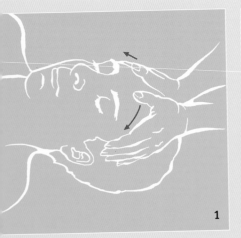

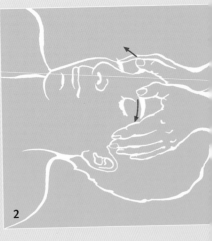

1 Place your hands on the sides of the head. Rest your thumbs on the temples. Apply pressure with your thumbs and rotate very slowly in a clockwise direction, completing at least ten circles. Check with your partner that the pressure is right. The slower you rotate, the more relaxing and effective it will be.

2 Ensure that your partner's eyes are closed. Bring your thumbs to the inner corners of the eyes, beside the nose, keeping them relaxed and straight. Very lightly, with no pressure whatsoever, glide your thumbs slowly across the eyelids. Do not drag the skin. Continue the movement down to the ears. Lift your hands, return to your original position and repeat.

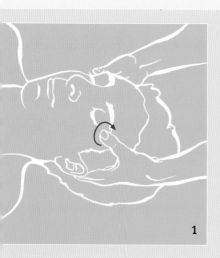

1

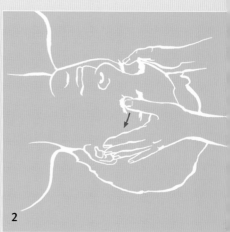

2

Place your thumbs either side of the top of the nose. Keep the other parts of your hands relaxed and in contact with the face to anchor the thumbs.

1 Glide the thumbs slowly down the sides of the nose to the nostrils. Keep the pressure light so you don't close the nose and inhibit breathing. Repeat. This time, keep your thumbs in place ready for the next stroke.

2 Keeping your thumbs in position, turn your hands so the fingers are anchored at the back of the neck. Press your thumbs into the face just outside each nostril. Apply pressure gradually and only to a depth that your partner is comfortable with. Hold for 10 seconds. If your partner has sinus congestion, repeat this step three times.

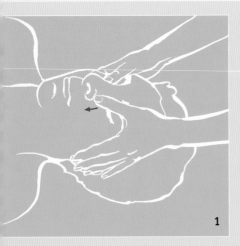

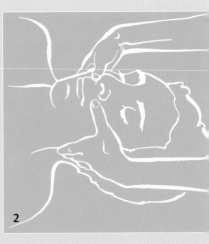

1

2

1 Place the pads of your three middle fingers underneath the cheekbones. Press slightly and very slowly rotate in a small circle. Lift the fingers just enough to move to the next section of cheekbone. Finish near the ears. Keep the pressure light unless your partner has a head cold or sinus congestion. In such cases, repeat three times.

2 Wrap your hands around the base of the head and position your thumbs on the ridge between the upper lip and nose. Lean your thumbs in slightly and glide them outwards to just beyond the edge of the upper lip, maintaining the pressure. Avoid dragging the skin and glide in a straight line rather than down towards the lips. Repeat twice.

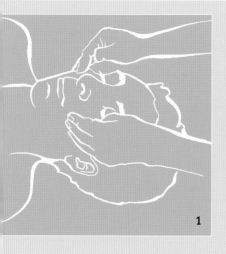

1

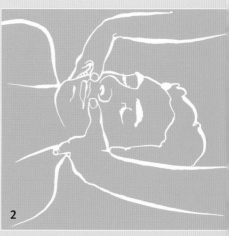

2

1  Position the thumbs along the ridge between the lower lip and the chin. Lean your thumbs in with slightly more pressure than you used in the previous step. Glide across the ridge in a straight line to just beyond the edge of the lower lip, keeping your pressure constant. Repeat twice.

2  Hook your fingers underneath the jaw, making sure they don't touch the throat. Secure them by placing your thumbs directly below the middle of the lips. Grasp the jaw firmly, but without causing any discomfort, and squeeze. As you do so, slowly rotate your thumbs in small circles. Keeping your hands firmly in place, move them outwards slightly along the jaw and repeat the rotation movement. Continue until you reach the ears. If your partner has a very tight or painful jaw, repeat twice.

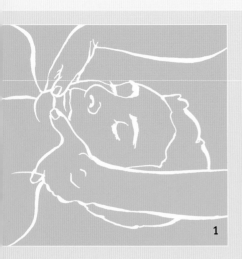
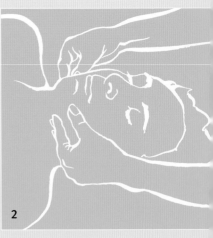

1

2

1 Smoothly move your hands to the ears. Wrap your fingers underneath the ears and place the heels of your hands on top to cover them. Very slowly, draw the hands down and off the ears. Don't stretch the skin as this may feel uncomfortable. Repeat once.

2 Rest one hand on the forehead and place the other on top. Lean in to apply slight pressure. Slowly release, then draw the hands back towards you. Repeat as soon as both hands are off the forehead.

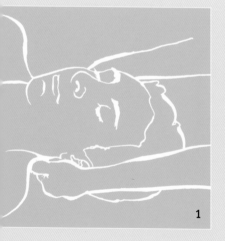

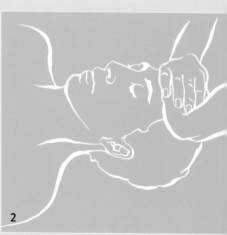

1 Place your hands around the sides of the face, lightly resting them on the cheeks. Maintain this gentle touch for 10 seconds. Keep your hands still and calm. You must be relaxed and breathing comfortably, as any tension will be noticeable and will transmit itself to your partner's face.

2 Slowly draw your hands back towards you, up the sides of the face. Keep your hands at an angle to the face so that only the edges make contact. Continue the movement, bringing your hands up onto the forehead, resting the thumbs in the centre.

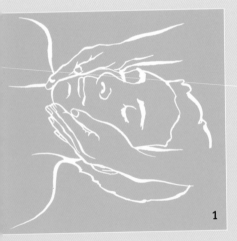

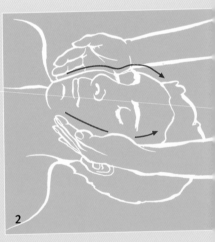

Position your thumbs alongside each other, in between the eyebrows. Your hands should be anchored on the sides of the head.

1 Inhale. As you exhale, lean forwards to put pressure on your thumbs. Slowly draw them straight back towards the hairline. You should be able to work quite deeply here, but quietly check with your partner what feels best.

2 Place one thumb on top of the other. Breathe in. As you breathe out, lean forwards, apply pressure to the head and hold for 5 seconds. Relax the thumbs and repeat, moving down the scalp as far as you can reach. It may help to imagine a line running down the centre of the head.

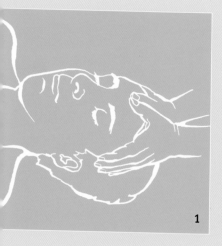

1

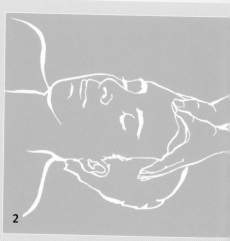

2

1  Bring your thumbs to rest either side of the 'line' you have just worked on. Breathe in. As you breathe out, lean into your thumbs. Lift them off briefly to reposition them. Continue to apply pressure in this way, moving down the scalp as far as you can reach.

2  Place the pads of your fingers on the head. Press into the scalp and rotate your fingers vigorously. If you find it difficult to maintain a rhythm with both hands, work with one at a time, resting the other on the head. Work thoroughly over the whole head, paying special attention to the area at the base of the skull.

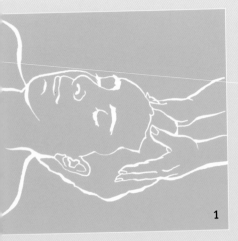

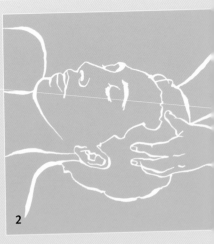

1

2

1   Place one hand on the head, with the back of the hand against the forehead. Draw the fingers slowly through the hair, then immediately repeat with the other hand. Keep the movement flowing, with your hands working in tandem. Work thoroughly on the entire head.

2   Slowly bring one hand to rest on the head. Place the other hand on top. Gradually lean your weight into your hands and the forehead. When you have reached a comfortable depth of pressure, maintain it for at least 10 seconds. Release the pressure very slowly so that your partner hardly notices what you're doing. Remove the top hand, then the bottom one. This movement should take at least 30 seconds.

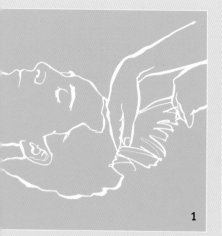

1

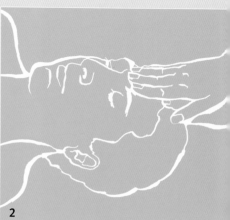

2

# arms and hands

The extent to which we express ourselves is revealed in our arms and hands. Holding our arms close to our body suggests that we are uneasy about taking up much space or asserting ourselves. Feelings and longings are, instead, buried in the belly and shoulders. The purpose of a good, sympathetic arm and hand treatment is to enable the suppressed individual to expand. We can all benefit from being more in touch with our arms and hands to express hidden or unspoken communication.

The arms sequence aims to encourage openness and the release of tension and blocked emotions. The hand massage can be given almost anywhere. As you can work directly on the skin without your partner having to remove any clothes, this is an ideal treatment for someone who is nervous of receiving massage or who is rarely touched. You will need very little oil; in fact, your partner may prefer you to use a favourite hand lotion. The skin on the hands is the thinnest on the body and is first to show signs of age. Increasing circulation to the area will contribute to keeping the hands healthy and youthful.

### The Muscles Explained

The deltoid muscle gives the shoulder its rounded contour and moves the arm away from the body. It inserts into the shaft of the humerus, the upper-arm bone. At its lower end, the humerus forms the elbow joint, which is moved by two main muscles: the biceps at the front and the triceps behind. The flexor and extensor muscles of the forearm also rise from the humerus and move the wrist and fingers. The brachioradialis muscle also stems from the humerus and inserts into the radius, which, like the ulna, is one of the forearm bones.

*Beneficial after recovery from a wrist or forearm fracture • Helps ease symptoms of lymphodema • Aids mobility in sufferers of tennis elbow*

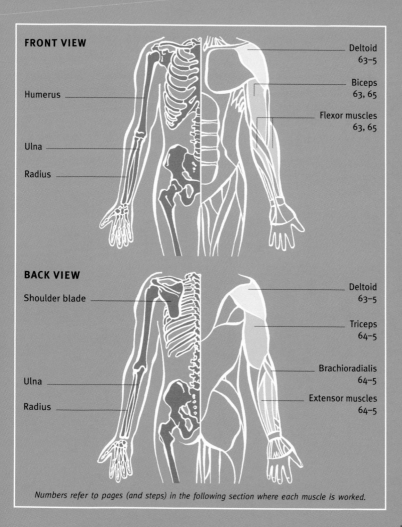

**FRONT VIEW**

Humerus

Ulna

Radius

Deltoid
63–5

Biceps
63, 65

Flexor muscles
63, 65

**BACK VIEW**

Shoulder blade

Ulna

Radius

Deltoid
63–5

Triceps
64–5

Brachioradialis
64–5

Extensor muscles
64–5

*Numbers refer to pages (and steps) in the following section where each muscle is worked.*

You should now have one hand on top of the arm and the other underneath.

Pull both hands slowly down the arm, over the hand and off. Take care to place your partner's hand on the floor gently.

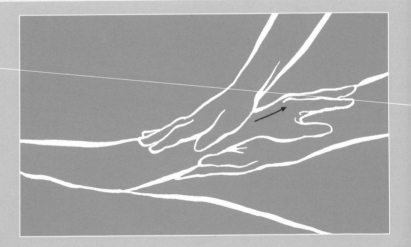

Cup your hands around the forearm, fingers pointing in opposite directions.

Glide your hands up the arm to the shoulder. Curve the upper hand around the shoulder and underneath the arm to draw both hands down the arm exactly as you did in the previous step.

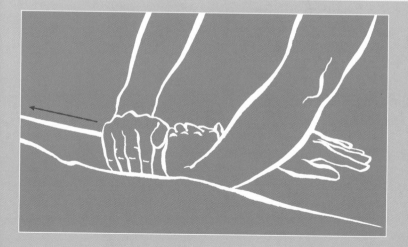

You need very little oil for the following hand strokes.

1  Hold your partner's hand in both your hands, leaving your thumbs free to work on the wrist. Use the ball of your thumbs to lean into the bony area of the wrist, and slowly rotate in between and over the bones. Work slowly and precisely in this way, all along the wrist.

2  Wrap your hands around your partner's hand, bringing the heels of your hands onto the back of their hand. Breathe in, and, as you breathe out, lean into your heels as they glide firmly across the hand in opposite directions. Return your hands to their original position and repeat the step.

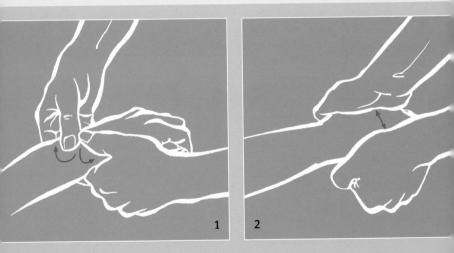

**Caution: Do not use this stroke on pregnant women – this area houses a powerful acupressure point for elimination.**

Wrap your fingers around your partner's palm leaving your thumbs free to work on the back of the hand.

1 Hold the hand firmly or rest it on your lap. Lean into and slowly rotate your thumbs in small circles over the back of the hand. Lift them off slightly at the end of each circle and move on to cover the rest of the back of the hand.

2 When you come to the web between the thumb and forefinger, lean your thumb into and circle this small area.

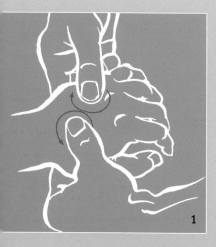

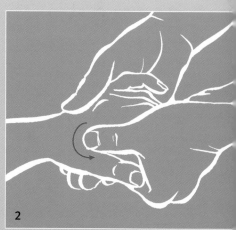

1  Insert your partner's thumb between your little finger and ring finger. Insert their little finger between the little finger and ring finger of your other hand. Pull the fingers slightly to stretch the palm.

2  Tuck your fingers under the back of their hand. Lean your thumbs in and rotate in small circles over the palm.

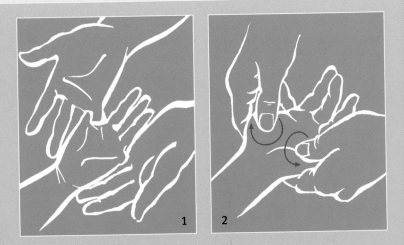

Hold your partner's hand in yours.

With your thumb on the back of their hand, lean it into the valley between the bones leading to the two smallest fingers. Glide along from the fingers to the wrist. Then repeat in the valleys between the other fingers.

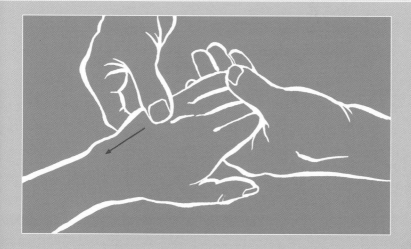

Clasp your partner's hand in yours.

Take hold of the base of the little finger between your thumb and forefinger. Squeeze it as your fingers slide firmly up to the tip. Here, squeeze and pinch the finger as you pull your fingers off.

Work along each finger in turn, ending on the thumb.

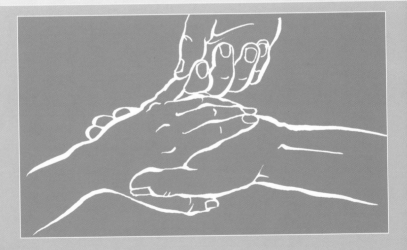

Hold your partner's forearm with one hand. Position your other hand under the forearm with the back of your hand against it.

1 Glide your hand along under the arm and hand.

2 Pull your hand up, inserting your fingers between your partner's fingers. Clasping them firmly with yours, pull your fingers up and back towards you. Repeat twice.

Repeat this entire sequence, from page 62, on the other arm and hand.

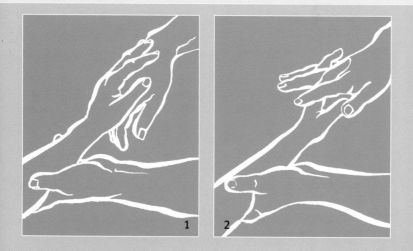

# fronts of legs and feet

The muscles in the fronts of the legs and the feet work extremely hard. We use them nearly all the time. Yet many of us misuse them, storing tension in the lower-leg area. This prevents force from being evenly distributed along the leg and can cause pain and discomfort. Massaging the calf mucles can ease this tension and bring feelings of deep relaxation to the recipient.

When working on the fronts of the legs, avoid applying direct pressure to the shinbone and the knee. Some people find the knee strokes uncomfortable, in which case use light effleurage around the knee instead. Working on the feet is doubly beneficial since you are, in effect, treating the entire body. The feet are covered with reflex areas that correspond to the organs and nerves, and as you work you will affect a much wider area than the feet alone. Prop up your partner's foot on a pillow so you can reach the sole of the foot easily. If they have ticklish feet, work firmly and apply extra pressure. If this doesn't help, it's usually best to stop, but to try again another day.

**The Muscles Explained**

The long bones of the legs – the femur, tibia and fibula – are crossed by large and powerful muscles. The upper end of the femur forms the hip joint with the hip bone, the ilium part of which can be felt by placing a hand on the hip. The fibula is a slender bone at the side of the tibia, which forms the lateral side of the ankle joint at its lower end. The quadriceps and the sartorius muscles lie on the front of the thigh and control extension of the patella (kneecap). The adductor muscles are found in the inner thigh area and work to stabilize the body during walking.

*Releases tension in the feet • Helps to repair ankle injuries*
*• Eases symptoms of water on the knee • Helps to relieve chilblains*

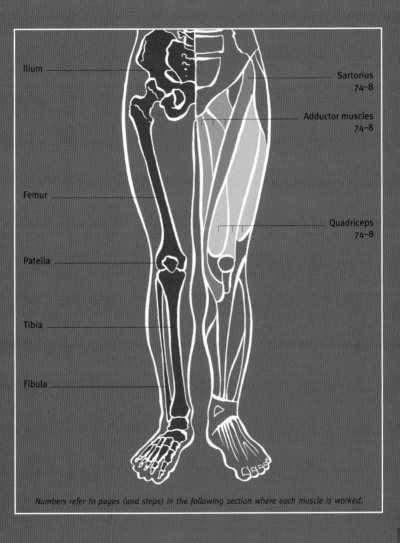

Ilium

Sartorius
74–8

Adductor muscles
74–8

Femur

Quadriceps
74–8

Patella

Tibia

Fibula

*Numbers refer to pages (and steps) in the following section where each muscle is worked.*

Kneel alongside your partner's ankles. Apply oil to your hands and make contact with the lower leg.

Inhale, and, as you exhale, lean into your hands, pushing them up the leg. Glide very lightly over the knee, using no pressure at all. As you approach the top of the leg, you may need to lean up on your knees to reach the entire length of the thigh, and to give you more body weight to drop into your stroke.

At the top of the thigh, curve your outside hand around the outside of the leg. Take your inside hand only as far up the leg as you feel is comfortable for your partner. Draw both hands back down the sides of the leg.

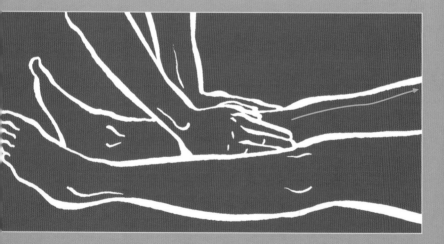

1 Cup your hands around the lower leg, your fingers pointing in opposite directions. Lean slightly into your hands without pressing down on the shinbone. Glide over the knee. Lean up on your knees and lean into the thigh. Curve your hands around the upper leg and draw them down the sides to the ankle.

2 Place your hands on the thigh just above the knee. Lean your weight into the thigh. To finish, draw your hands back to the knee.

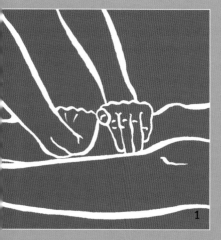

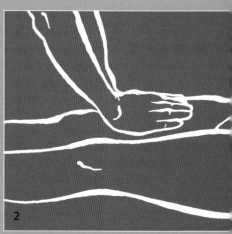

1  Change your position so that you are kneeling facing your partner's upper leg. Place your hands side by side on the thigh. Lean into one hand and pick up and squeeze the flesh and muscle between your fingers and thumb. Push towards your other hand as it begins the same movement. Continue slowly and rhythmically.

2  Reposition yourself so that you're kneeling alongside your partner's knees. Place both hands just above the knee, heels together and fingers wrapped around the sides of the leg. Inhale and, as you exhale, lean into the heels of your hands and push them firmly towards your fingers. Repeat the stroke, moving up the leg, until you've covered the entire thigh. Bring your hands back to the starting position and repeat the movement with one hand at a time, resting your other hand on the leg.

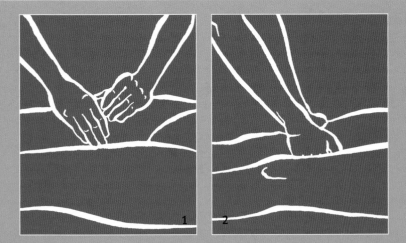

Turn back to face your partner's upper leg again. Place both hands flat on the thigh, fingers pointing away from you.

Inhale and, as you exhale, lean in and push one hand slowly and firmly across the thigh, then pull the other hand slowly back towards you.

Use your body weight to bring impact to your hands and make sure that you're lifting up flesh and muscle as the hands criss-cross against each other – not merely sliding the hands over the skin. This needs to be a dynamic, deep and thorough movement.

Continue this action until you have covered the whole thigh.

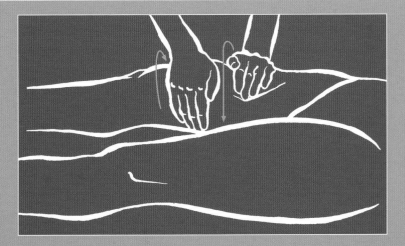

Change position to kneel alongside your partner's knees again. Place both hands flat on the leg just above the knee.

1  Inhale. Exhale and lean into the heels of your hands. Push them, one at a time, up the centre of the thigh to the top. Keep your fingers soft, relaxed and in contact with the leg. Repeat on the outer and inner thigh, starting at the knee each time. Keep the momentum slow, deep and thorough.

2  Form your hands into loose fists and place them just above the knee. Lean in slightly and push your knuckles, one after the other, up to the top of the thigh. Return to the starting position and repeat the movement up the inner and outer thigh. The latter can be very sensitive, so increase the pressure gradually and be aware of your partner's response.

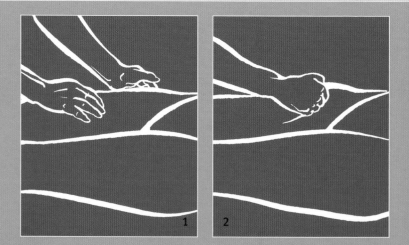

1  Wrap your hands under the knee, leaving your thumbs available to work around the joint. Beginning at the top of the knee, lean your thumbs gradually into the grooves around the outside of the kneepad. Work outwards from the top of the knee, around the sides, and follow the joint round to the bottom. Apply pressure slowly and only to a depth that your partner finds comfortable. Press towards the centre of the knee, and maintain constant pressure for 5 seconds at each indentation.

2  Rest one hand on the leg below the knee. Place your other hand on the knee and, with your thumb, lean into the grooves and indentations that you worked on in the previous stroke, but this time rotate your thumb in slow circles instead of pressing in.

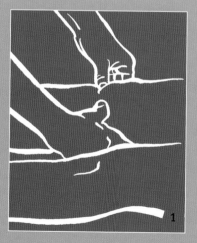

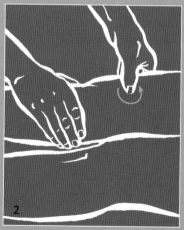

Kneel at your partner's feet. Apply more oil to your hands.

1 Gently cup your hands around the foot and ankle, fingers pointing in opposite directions. Avoid pulling the foot or applying any pressure at this point. Inhale, and, as you exhale, glide your hands up sideways over the foot and onto the lower leg.

2 Turn your hands around to pull back towards yourself, gliding your upper hand underneath the foot and turning your lower one onto the foot. As you pull your hands back towards you, lean back slightly to give the movement impact.

Repeat three times.

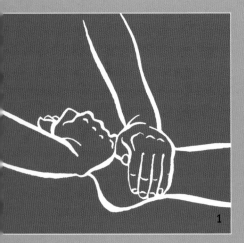

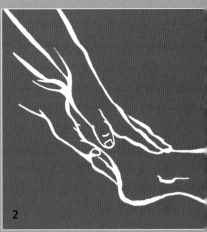

1 Place one hand flat on the sole of the foot, with the heel of your hand fitting securely into the instep. Hold the ankle firmly with your other hand. Breathe in, and, as you breathe out, lean forwards to push your hand gradually into the foot, towards your partner's knee. Hold the stretch for 10 seconds and repeat.

2 Place one hand on top of the leg, just above the ankle, and wrap your other hand securely around the top of the foot. Breathe in, and, as you breathe out, lean into the hand on the foot to gradually stretch the foot downwards. Be careful to apply the stretch slowly and ask your partner to tell you when the stretch is sufficient. Repeat once.

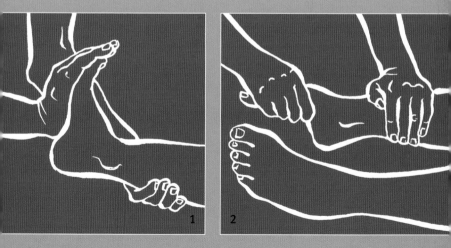

1   Wrap your hands around the sides of the foot. The heels of your
    hands should rest next to each other on top. To achieve this position,
    sit upright over the foot with your arms straight. Lean into the heels
    of your hands to glide them firmly across the foot in opposite
    directions. Continue until you have covered the whole foot.

2   Hold the base of the foot firmly in one hand. Make your other hand
    into a fist and place it on top of the foot. Rotate your fingers around
    to make small circular movements with your knuckles. Work slowly
    and thoroughly all over the top of the foot. Repeat twice.

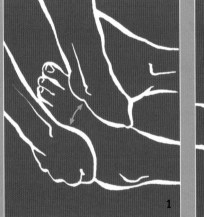
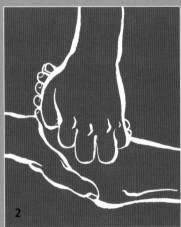

1 Wrap both hands around the foot and place your thumbs on the top. Lean your thumbs in and slowly rotate them in small circles. Work evenly over the top of the foot and around the anklebone itself. Keep your thumbs straight and relaxed. Cover the foot in this way three times.

2 Hold the heel firmly with one hand. Wrap the other hand around the top of the foot so your thumb rests on the sole. Press your thumb into the foot and slowly rotate in a small circle. Repeat until you have thoroughly covered the entire sole of the foot.

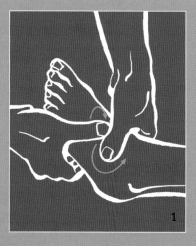

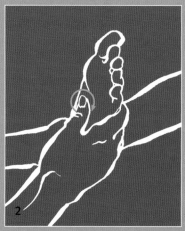

You may find that placing a pillow under your partner's foot makes these steps more comfortable for you.

1  Wrap both hands around the front of the foot to leave your thumbs free to work on the sole. The thumbs should be next to each other. Breathe in, and, as you breathe out, lean into the tops of your thumbs to glide firmly across the foot in opposite directions. Extend the stroke right out to the edges of the foot. Repeat until you've covered the sole of the foot.

2  Hold the foot securely around the ankle with one hand. Make your other hand into a fist and rotate your knuckles slowly over the sole of the foot, exactly as you did on the top of the foot. Continue around the ankle and the sides of the foot. Repeat.

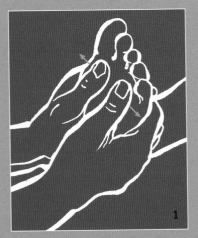
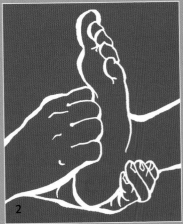

1   Hold the foot with one hand. Clasp the sides of the big toe between your finger and thumb and squeeze firmly. Pull the toe gently as you move your finger and thumb up and off. If your partner finds this ticklish, try to be firmer and more assertive in your touch. Repeat on each of the toes, making sure to begin at the webs of the toes and to squeeze the sides rather than the top and bottom of each toe.

2   Wrap your hands around the foot, fingers pointing in opposite directions. Glide your hands over the foot up onto the lower leg. Turn the hands around to glide one hand underneath the foot and the other on top. Repeat three times and, on the final stroke, hold the foot for 30 seconds to 'ground' your partner.

Repeat this entire sequence, from page 74, on the front of the other leg and foot.

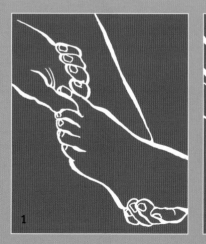

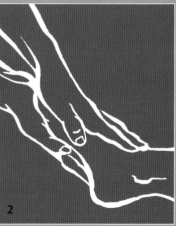

# stimulating massage

## 30-MINUTE SEQUENCE

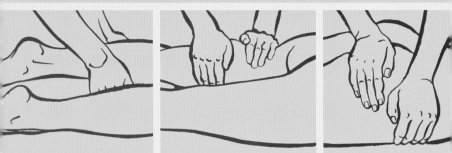

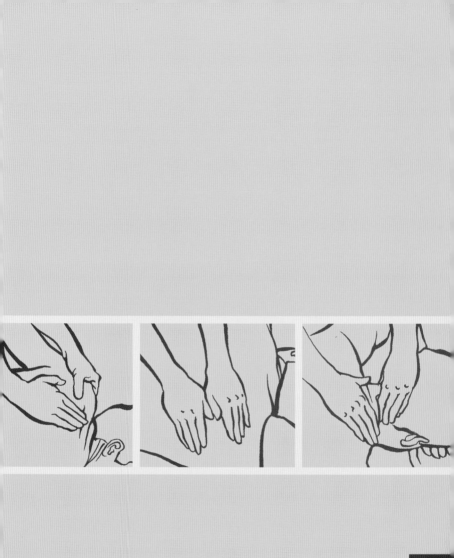

Place your hands on the lower leg, in a cupped position, with your fingers pointing in opposite directions.

Breathe in, and, as you breathe out, lean gently into your hands, gliding them slowly up the leg. Ease the pressure as you reach the back of the knee, then reapply once you've cleared the sensitive area. Maintain the cupped position as you glide onto the thigh, and sweep firmly around the buttock with your outside hand.

Complete the stroke by drawing both hands lightly down the leg to the ankle.

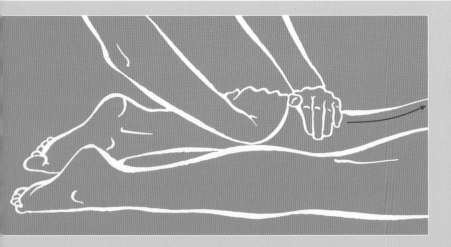

**Caution: Avoid petrissage, kneading and wringing strokes if your partner has varicose veins.**

Here, you are using a wringing motion to squeeze tension and trapped toxins out of the muscles.

Reposition yourself to face your partner's calf.

Wrap your hands around the calf, embracing the muscles between your thumb and fingers. Use a firm wringing movement to lift and twist the muscles. Work over the entire calf.

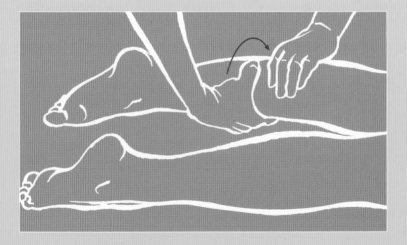

Facing your partner's thigh, place your hands parallel on the lower thigh.

Push your hands in opposite directions, then back again. Make this wringing action dynamic, lifting and squeezing the muscle. Work up the thigh.

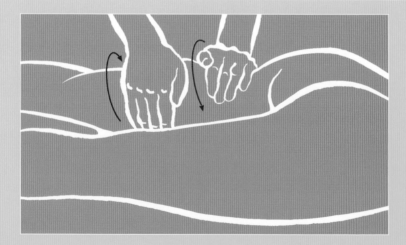

Place both hands on the calf just above the ankle, the heels of your hands next to each other, fingers wrapped around the front of the leg.

Breathe in, and, as you breathe out, lean into the heels of your hands, pushing them away from each other and off the leg. Repeat this stroke, moving up the calf until you reach the knee.

Reduce the pressure as you pass over the knee, then continue to work all the way up to the thigh.

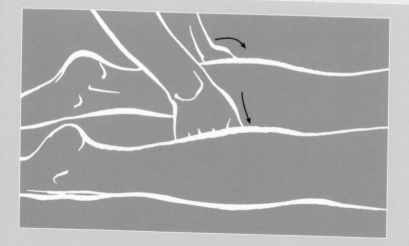

Form your hands into relaxed fists and rest them on the thigh.

Leaning slightly into your hands, run your knuckles up the inside of the thigh, one hand after the other. Don't work too far up. Repeat on the centre of the thigh. Work up to the buttock, then bring your hands back to the starting position to repeat.

Gradually bring your hands around to the outside. This area can be quite sensitive, so work lightly to begin with, slowly increasing the depth of pressure. But, as you move onto the buttock, really lean in deeply.

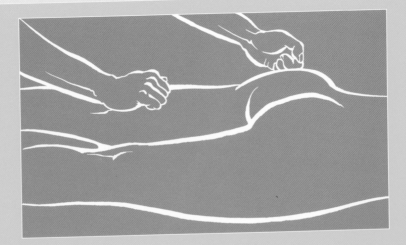

Move around your partner's body so that the leg and buttock you have been working on are furthest from you.

Lean up on your knees. Still working on the same side, place both hands flat on the buttock.

Inhale, and, as you exhale, push into the buttock, squeezing the flesh and muscle between the heel of your hand and your fingers. Repeat with the other hand. Work rhythmically, completing the movement at least five times with each hand.

Repeat the steps shown on pages 88–93 on the other leg.

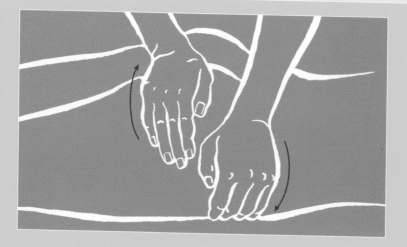

Apply the oil to your hands, away from your partner's body. Breathe in, and, as you breathe out, make contact.

1  Effleurage by gliding both hands firmly up the back and around the shoulders.

2  Draw the hands lightly down the sides of the back to the starting position.

The dynamic here is on the upward motion towards the heart with light contact on the return stroke. Lean your body into your hands to apply more pressure. You can come up on your knees but keep the pressure steady. Repeat this four or five times.

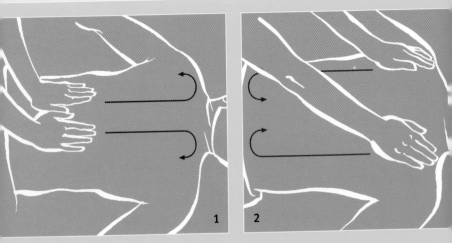

Glide your hands up the back once again.

1 Extend your hands over the shoulders, hook the fingers into the front of the shoulder muscles and pull back, leaning your body back for maximum effect.

2 The return stroke uses only the sides of the hands for very light contact, with the hands opened out.

Repeat twice.

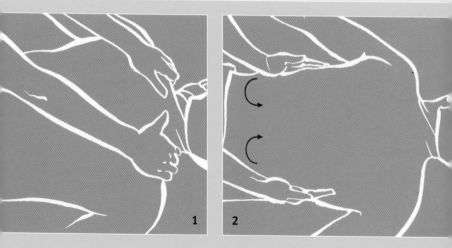

Place your hands on the lower back as if you are beginning to effleurage.

Push your hands out to the sides of the body, circling them around and back to meet each other. Continue the stroke, moving up the back with each set of circles until you reach the shoulders.

Draw the hands down to the lower back, using the sides of your hands, as on page 95.

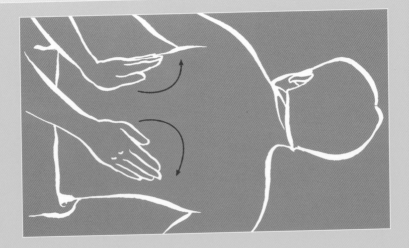

Move yourself round so that your knees are facing the shoulder blade opposite.

1 Effleurage by placing both hands on the shoulder blade and pushing down towards the arm. Glide your hands in the direction of the arrows. Use your body weight to give momentum. When you push over the shoulder blade, come up onto your knees if necessary, but only if you can still control the pressure. Lean backwards using your full body weight when you pull the hands back.

2 To finish, rest your hands in opposite directions at the top of the shoulder blade.

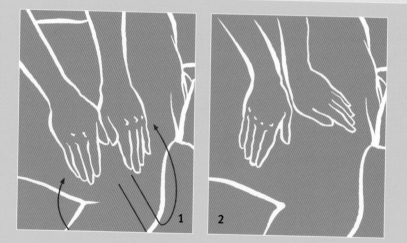

Place your hands on the lower back, fingers facing away from each other.

1  Lean the heels of your hands into the groove either side of the spine and begin to push towards your fingers. Do not allow the fingers to glide down the back. Work up the back to the shoulder blades, reducing the pressure as you cover the kidney area.

2  Repeat the stroke, working on one side of the spine at a time. Keep your hands parallel; rest one while the other works. You should work on the side furthest from you, so move round to the other side when you've finished one half. Work up to the shoulder blades.

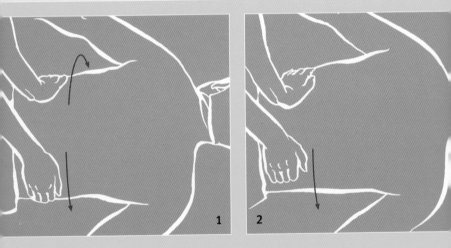

Come up onto your knees. Anchor your hand by wrapping your fingers around the front of the shoulder.

1 Push the heel of the hand into the muscle until the hand slips off the shoulder. Use your full body weight to push into and squeeze the muscle. Repeat five times using both hands alternately.

2 Support yourself with one hand and, with the other, hold the shoulder muscle between the fingers and thumb. Lean in, squeeze firmly and push the thumb and the heel of your hand right off the shoulder. Repeat with the other hand. Complete this step five times with each hand.

Move round to the other side of your partner's body and repeat both steps on the other shoulder.

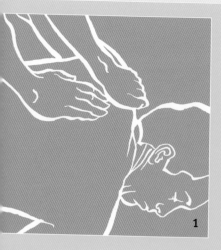
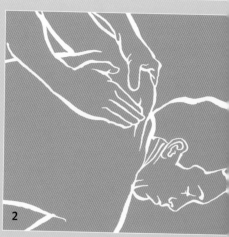

Ask your partner to rest their head on their hands. Position yourself comfortably with your body weight over the neck and head. Try placing your outside leg in front of you, foot parallel to your partner's head, inside leg kneeling up.

1   Stabilize the head with one hand while the other squeezes into the neck, working up towards the base of the skull. Don't let your thumb and forefinger slip around to the throat. Work up and down the neck three times.

2   Squeeze down the neck with one hand as the other squeezes up to meet it. Use your thumb and fingertips rather than the whole hand. Work up and down the neck three times.

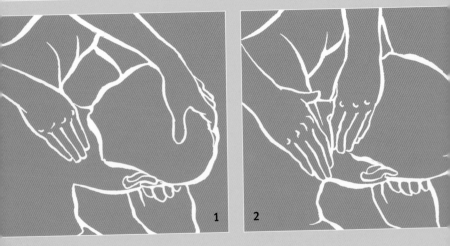

Place both hands on the upper back.

While one hand rests, pull the other back firmly towards your partner's head and around the edge of the shoulder blade in the direction of the arrow. Push the heel of your hand into and along the shoulder muscle, out to the arm. Repeat the stroke on the other side.

You can also do this stroke using both hands at once.

To complete the treatment, cover your partner with a towel and leave them to relax for a few minutes.

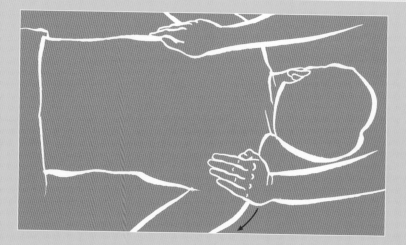

# de-stress massage

## 30-MINUTE SEQUENCE

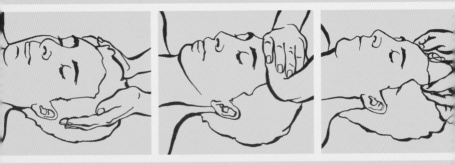

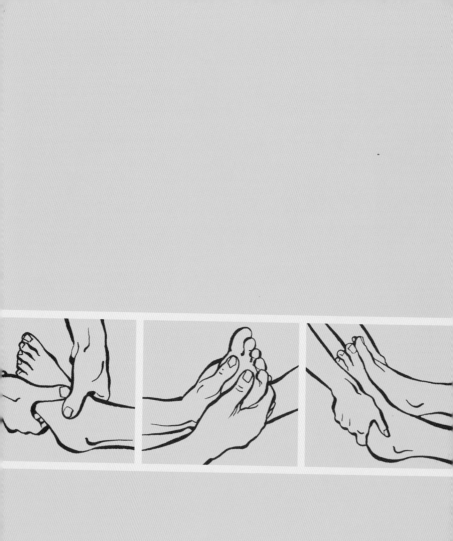

Kneel astride your partner's head. If your hands are dry, apply half a teaspoon of oil.

1  Gently place your hands on the sides of your partner's head. Stay in this position for about 20 seconds, breathing in and out slowly and deeply. This will help you to relax and will ease you into your massage.

2  Move your hands forwards and rest them on the forehead very gradually and deliberately. Position the thumbs and the heels of your hands in the centre of the forehead and wrap your fingers around the sides. Maintain a firm pressure without actually pressing into your hands. Be careful not to push the forehead down towards the eyebrows. Hold for at least 20 seconds.

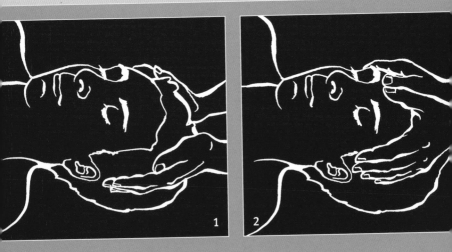

1  Inhale. Exhale and lean forwards slightly, transferring your weight into your thumbs. Glide them towards the ears, keeping them relaxed but straight, using even pressure along their entire length. When you reach the ears, place your thumbs back on the forehead, just above the original position. Repeat, moving upwards each time until you reach the hairline.

2  Rest the thumbs on the eyebrows. Inhale. Exhale and lean forwards to transfer weight into your thumbs. Draw them slowly across the eyebrows and down to the ears. Lift the hands, return to your starting position and repeat. Ask your partner what amount of pressure they find comfortable.

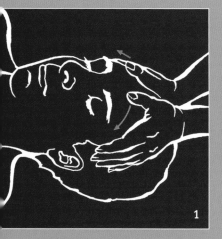

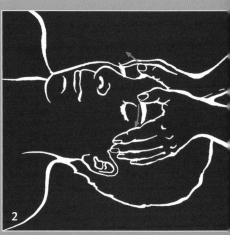

1  Place your hands on the sides of the head. Rest your thumbs on the temples. Apply pressure with your thumbs and rotate very slowly in a clockwise direction, completing at least ten circles. Check with your partner that the pressure is right. The slower you rotate, the more relaxing and effective it will be.

2  Keeping your hands in position, place one thumb on top of the other and slowly rest them on the area just above the centre of the eyebrows. Apply firm but gentle pressure to the forehead. Maintain for 20 seconds, then slowly release.

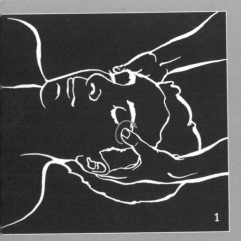

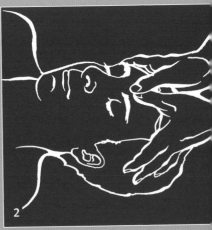

1 Slowly bring one hand to rest on the head. Place the other hand on top. Gradually lean your weight into your hands and the forehead. When you have reached a comfortable depth of pressure, maintain it for at least 10 seconds. Release the pressure very slowly so that your partner hardly notices what you're doing. Remove the top hand, then the bottom one. This movement should take at least 30 seconds.

2 Using the pads of your fingers, stroke lightly and slowly from the eyebrows to the hairline, one hand after the other. Cover the whole forehead in this way.

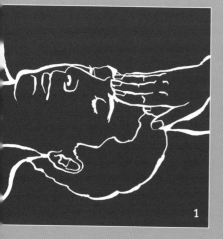

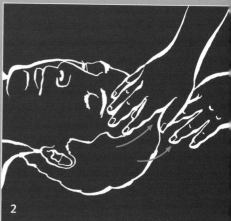

Place your right hand on the forehead and your left hand directly on top. Interlock your fingers and spread them across the forehead.

Using the pads of your fingers, apply firm pressure for a count of 30.

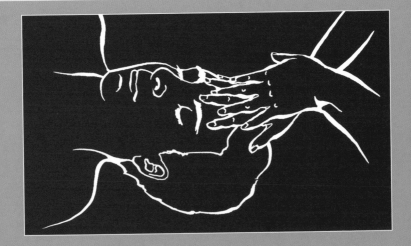

1 Rest one hand on the forehead and place the other on top. Lean in to apply slight pressure. Slowly release, then draw the hands back towards you. Repeat as soon as both hands are off the forehead.

2 Using two fingers of each hand, apply the pads to either side of the head, just in front of the top of the ears. Slowly circle over the area several times.

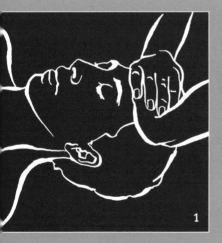

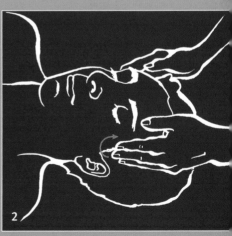

Position your thumbs alongside each other, in between the eyebrows. Your hands should be anchored on the sides of the head.

1  Inhale. As you exhale, lean forwards to put pressure on your thumbs. Slowly draw them straight back towards the hairline. You should be able to work quite deeply here, but quietly check with your partner what feels best.

2  Place one thumb on top of the other. Breathe in. As you breathe out, lean forwards, apply pressure to the head and hold for 5 seconds. Relax the thumbs and repeat, moving down the scalp as far as you can reach. It may help to imagine a line running down the centre of the head.

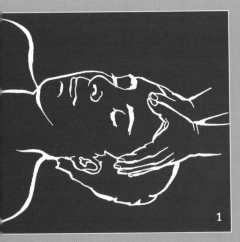

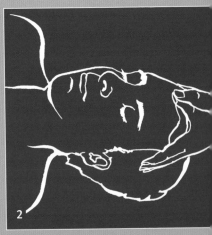

1 Bring your thumbs to rest either side of the 'line' you have just worked on. Breathe in. As you breathe out, lean into your thumbs. Lift them off briefly to reposition them. Continue to apply pressure in this way, moving down the scalp as far as you can reach.

2 Place the pads of your fingers on the head. Press into the scalp and rotate your fingers vigorously. If you find it difficult to maintain a rhythm with both hands, work with one at a time, resting the other on the head. Work thoroughly over the whole head, paying special attention to the area at the base of the skull.

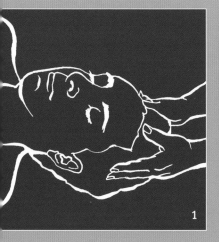

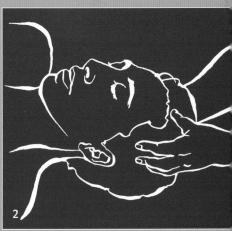

1  Place one hand on the head, with the back of the hand against the forehead. Draw the fingers slowly through the hair, then immediately repeat with the other hand. Keep the movement flowing, with both hands working in tandem. Work thoroughly on the entire head.

2  With your thumb and forefinger, gently tug a small tuft of hair on the hairline. Pull firmly so that the forehead moves. Work rhythmically, pulling first on one side and then the other. Move along the hairline from above the ears to the centre of the head. This movement is tremendous for releasing tension and worry lines in the forehead.

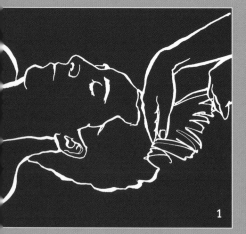

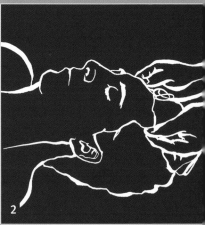

Once you have finished working on the forehead, move round your partner's side. Using your hands alternately, slowly brush down the body until you reach the feet.

This is a wonderful way of moving from one area of the body to another without loosing contact.

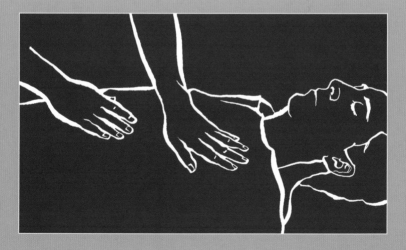

Kneel at your partner's feet. Apply oil to your hands.

1 Gently cup your hands around the foot and ankle, fingers pointing in opposite directions. Avoid pulling the foot or applying any pressure at this point. Inhale, and, as you exhale, glide your hands up sideways over the foot and onto the lower leg.

2 Turn your hands around to pull back towards yourself, gliding your upper hand underneath the foot and turning your lower one onto the foot. As you pull your hands back towards you, lean back slightly to give the movement impact.

Repeat three times.

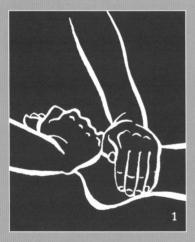
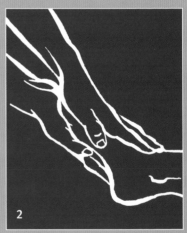

1 Wrap your hands around the sides of the foot. The heels of your hands should rest next to each other on top. To achieve this position, sit upright over the foot with your arms straight. Lean into the heels of your hands to glide them firmly across the foot in opposite directions. Continue until you have covered the whole foot.

2 Hold the base of the foot firmly in one hand. Make your other hand into a fist and place it on top of the foot. Rotate your fingers around to make small circular movements with your knuckles. Work slowly and thoroughly all over the top of the foot. Repeat twice.

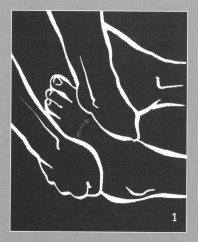

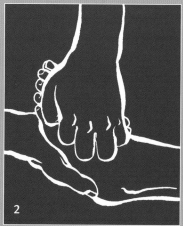

1 Wrap both hands around the foot and place your thumbs on the top. Lean your thumbs in and slowly rotate them in small circles. Work evenly over the top of the foot and around the anklebone itself. Keep your thumbs straight and relaxed. Cover the foot in this way three times.

2 Hold the heel firmly with one hand. Wrap the other hand around the top of the foot so your thumb rests on the sole. Press your thumb into the foot and slowly rotate in a small circle. Repeat until you have thoroughly covered the entire sole of the foot.

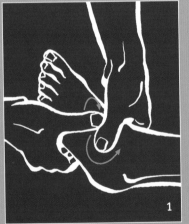
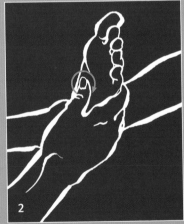

You may find that placing a pillow under your partner's foot makes these steps more comfortable for you.

1   Wrap both hands around the front of the foot to leave your thumbs free to work on the sole. The thumbs should be next to each other. Breathe in, and, as you breathe out, lean into the tops of your thumbs to glide firmly across the foot in opposite directions. Extend the stroke right out to the edges of the foot. Repeat until you've covered the sole of the foot.

2   Hold the foot securely around the ankle with one hand. Make your other hand into a fist and rotate your knuckles slowly over the sole of the foot, exactly as you did on the top of the foot. Continue around the ankle and the sides of the foot. Repeat.

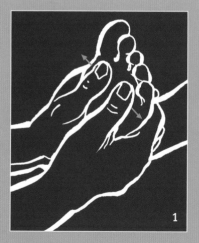

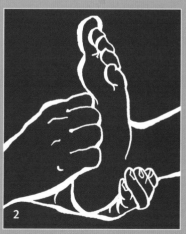

1 Hold the foot with one hand. Clasp the sides of the big toe between your finger and thumb and squeeze firmly. Pull the toe gently as you move your finger and thumb up and off. If your partner finds this ticklish, try to be firmer and more assertive in your touch. Repeat on each of the toes, making sure to begin at the webs of the toes and to squeeze the sides rather than the top and bottom of each toe.

2 Wrap your hands around the foot, fingers pointing in opposite directions. Glide your hands over the foot up onto the lower leg. Turn the hands around to glide one hand underneath the foot and the other on top. Repeat three times.

Repeat all the strokes shown on pages 114–18 on the other foot.

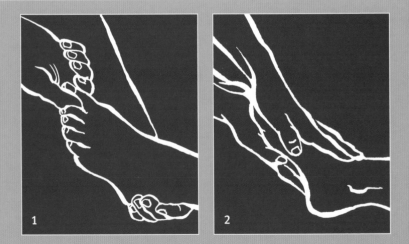

Hold both the feet around the sides. Give them a gentle squeeze, then maintain the contact restfully for at least 30 seconds.

This is a great way to end the treatment and will help your partner to feel more grounded.

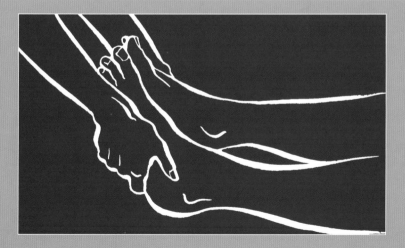

# soothing hand massage

## 20-MINUTE SEQUENCE

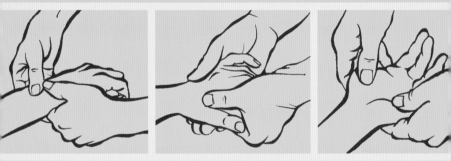

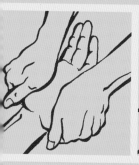
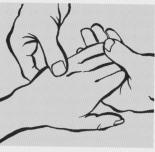
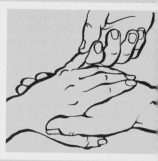

You need very little oil for the following hand strokes.

1 Hold your partner's hand in both your hands, leaving your thumbs free to work on the wrist. Use the ball of your thumbs to lean into the bony area of the wrist, and slowly rotate in between and over the bones. Work slowly and precisely in this way, all along the wrist.

2 Wrap your hands around your partner's hand, bringing the heels of your hands onto the back of their hand. Breathe in, and, as you breathe out, lean into your heels as they glide firmly across the hand in opposite directions. Return your hands to their original position and repeat the step.

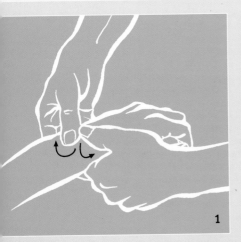

1

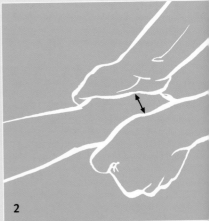

2

**Caution: Do not use this stroke on pregnant women – this area houses a powerful acupressure point for elimination.**

Wrap your fingers around your partner's palm, leaving your thumbs free to work on the back of the hand.

1 Hold the hand firmly or rest it on your lap. Lean into and slowly rotate your thumbs in small circles over the back of the hand. Lift them off slightly at the end of each circle and move on to cover the rest of the back of the hand.

2 When you come to the web between the thumb and forefinger, lean your thumb into and circle this small area.

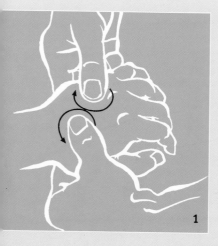

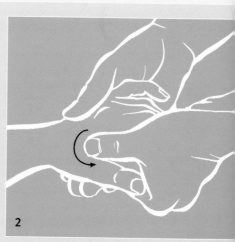

1 Insert your partner's thumb between your little finger and ring finger. Insert their little finger between the little finger and ring finger of your other hand. Pull the fingers slightly to stretch the palm.

2 Tuck your fingers under the back of their hand. Lean your thumbs in and rotate in small circles over the palm.

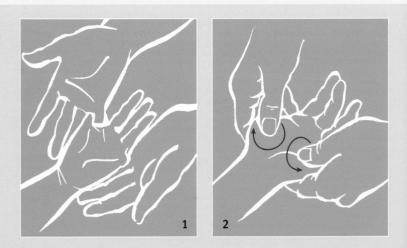

Wrap your hands around your partner's hand, placing the heels of your hands on the centre of their palm. Using slow, firm pressure, glide the heels, in opposite directions, out across the palm.

Return your hands to the original position and repeat the stroke.

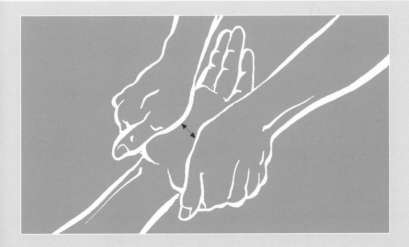

Hold your partner's hand in yours.

1 With your thumb on the back of their hand, lean it into the valley between the bones leading to the two smallest fingers. Glide along from the fingers to the wrist. Then repeat in the valleys between the other fingers.

2 Take hold of the base of the little finger between your thumb and forefinger. Squeeze it as your fingers slide firmly up to the tip. Here, squeeze and pinch the finger as you pull your fingers off. Work along each finger in turn, ending on the thumb.

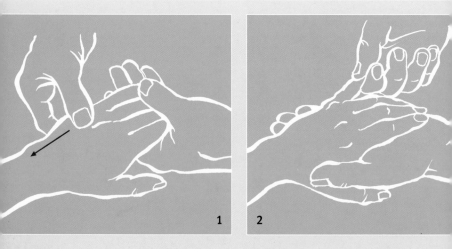

Hold your partner's hand in your inside hand. With your other hand, gently squeeze the wrist between your thumb and fingers, and slowly move up the arm to the shoulder. Then continue the movement back down to the starting position. Repeat the stroke 2–3 times.

Repeat this entire sequence, from page 122, on the other hand.

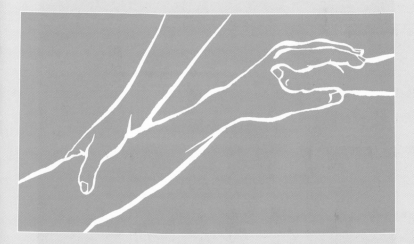

## ABOUT THE AUTHOR

**Fiona Harrold** studied and taught massage for many years before founding The London College of Massage in 1987. Her published works include: *The Massage Manual*; *Therapy Cards: Massage*; *Massage Cures*; and an instructional video demonstrating her techniques. She is now a leading life coach, and is dedicated to helping people from all walks of life discover their own true qualities and talents. Fiona is the author of the bestselling *Be Your Own Life Coach*, as well as *The 10-Minute Life Coach*, *Reinvent Yourself* and *The Seven Roles of Success*. She appears regularly on television and in newspapers and magazines. Visit Fiona's website at fionaharrold.com.

## ABOUT THE CONSULTANT

**Marc Salnicki** is a director of The London College of Massage and has practised and taught massage for many years. For massage courses and treatments, contact The London College of Massage on 020 3259 0000, or visit the website at www.massagelondon.com.